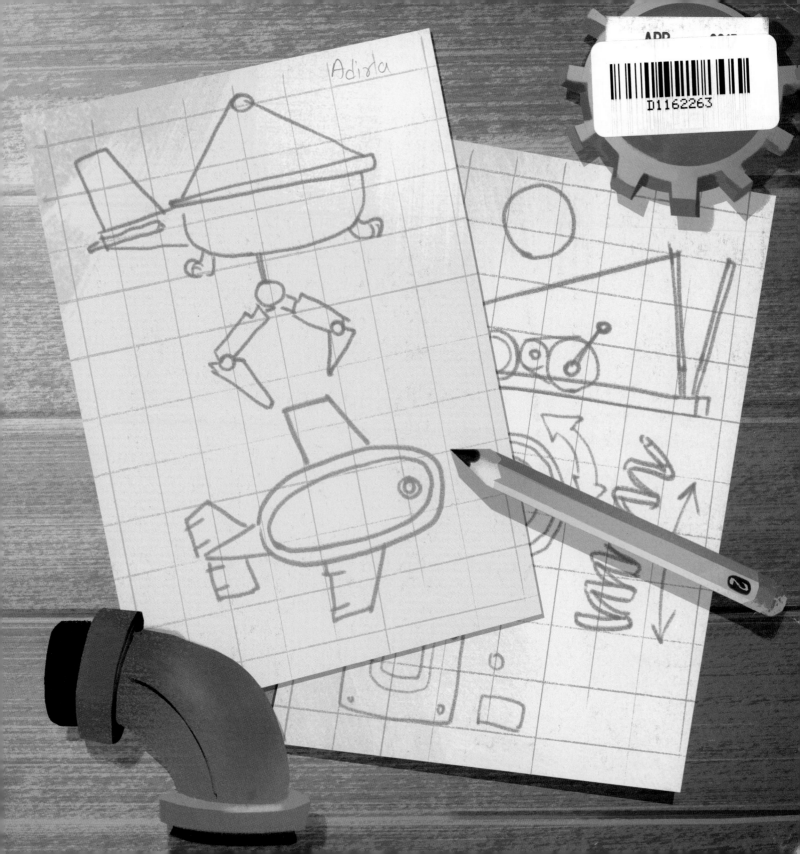

BOATS BUILT FOR SPEED with Davey and Pearl

Copyright © 2016 Green Toys Inc.

Art Direction & Storyboards by Brian Gulassa
Additional Art by Lawrence Cruz
Book Design by Iain R. Morris
Produced by Cameron + Company
www.cameronbooks.com

ISBN: 978-0-9971434-1-6
Lot# 1222150509
SKU# BKBT-4341

Printed in the USA

Green Toys Inc.
4000 Bridgeway, Suite 100
Sausalito, CA 94965
www.greentoys.com

BOATS BUILT FOR SPEED

with Davey and Pearl

Written by Robert von Goeben

Illustrated by Mike Yamada

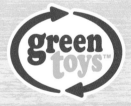

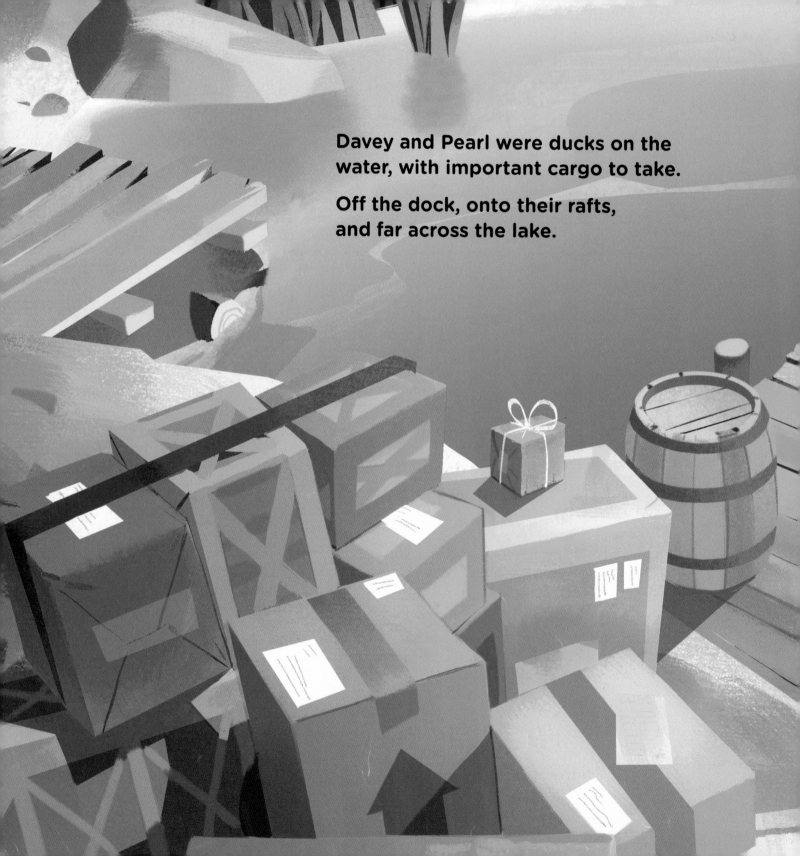

Davey and Pearl were ducks on the water, with important cargo to take.

Off the dock, onto their rafts, and far across the lake.

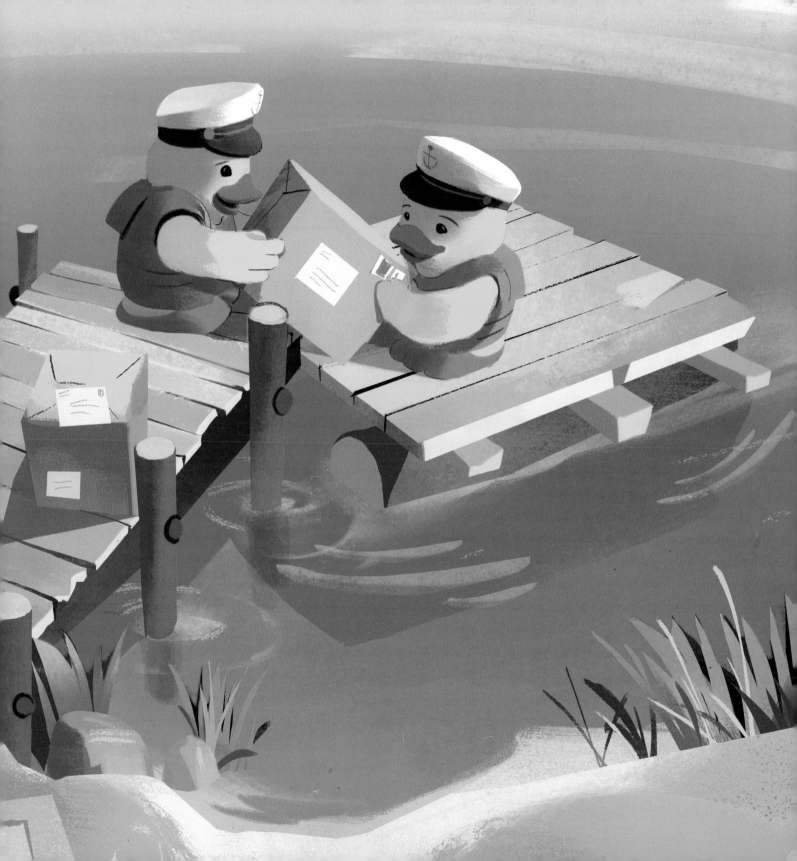

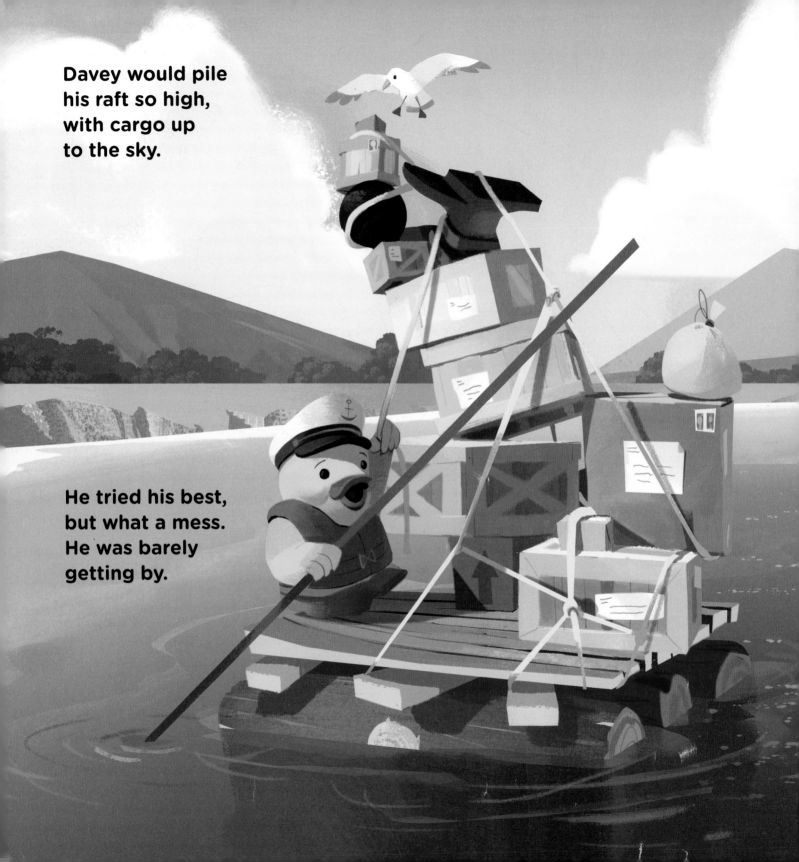

Davey would pile
his raft so high,
with cargo up
to the sky.

He tried his best,
but what a mess.
He was barely
getting by.

Pearl, however, was calm and cool,
and always thought it through.

She packed her cargo carefully,
her limit she always knew.

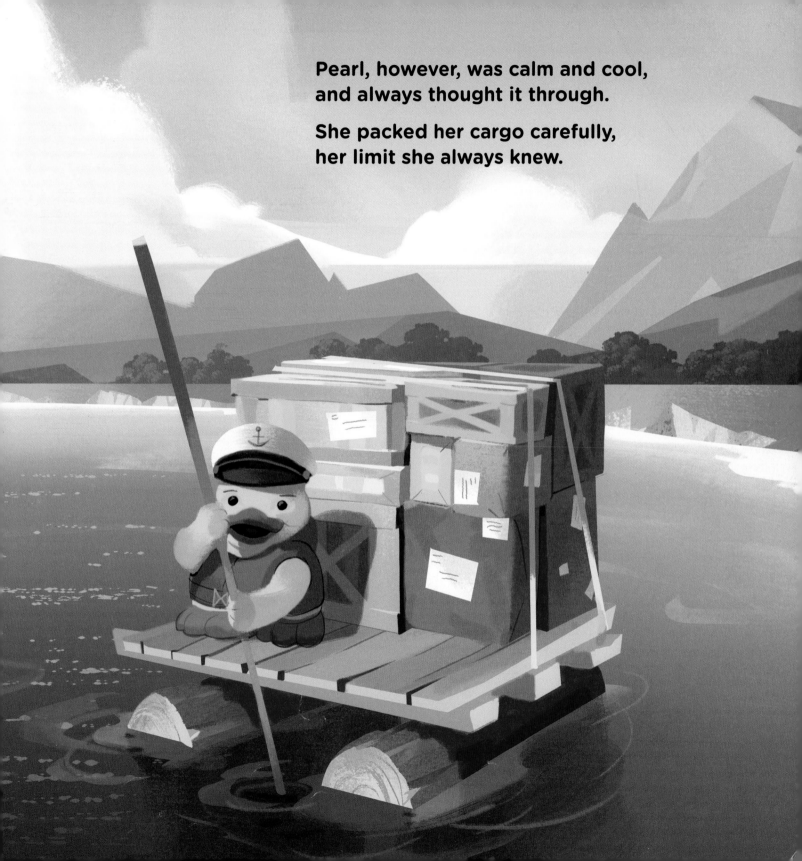

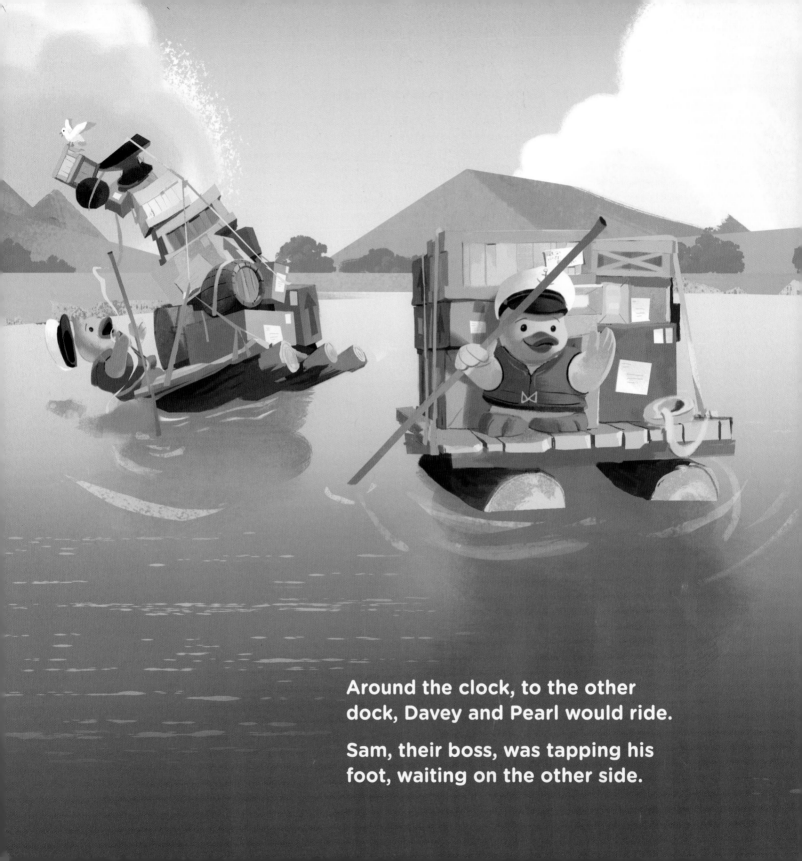

Around the clock, to the other dock, Davey and Pearl would ride.

Sam, their boss, was tapping his foot, waiting on the other side.

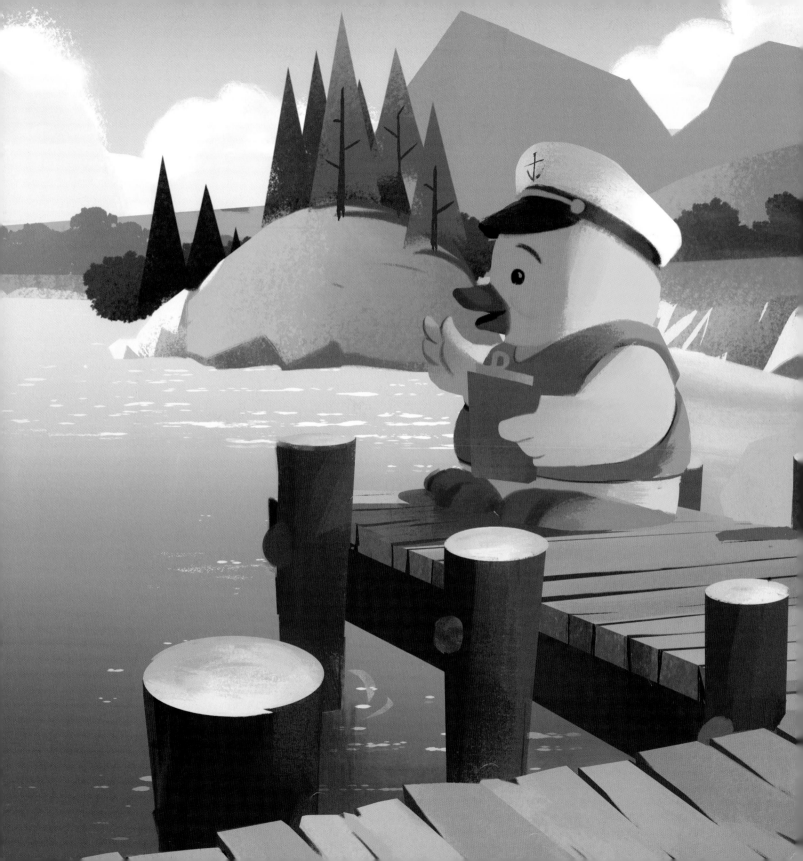

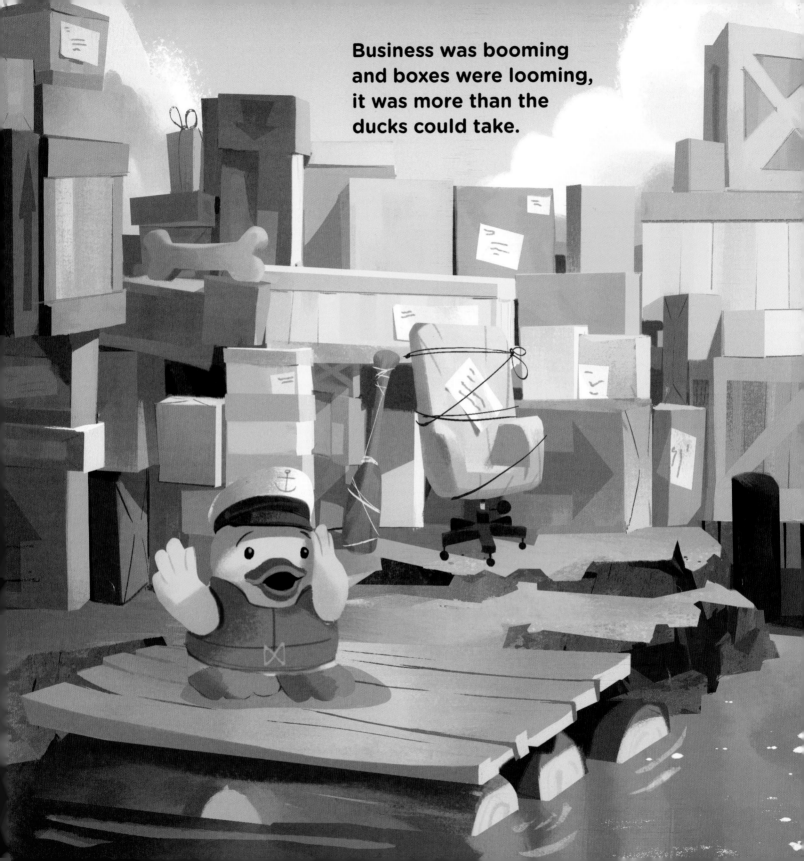

Business was booming
and boxes were looming,
it was more than the
ducks could take.

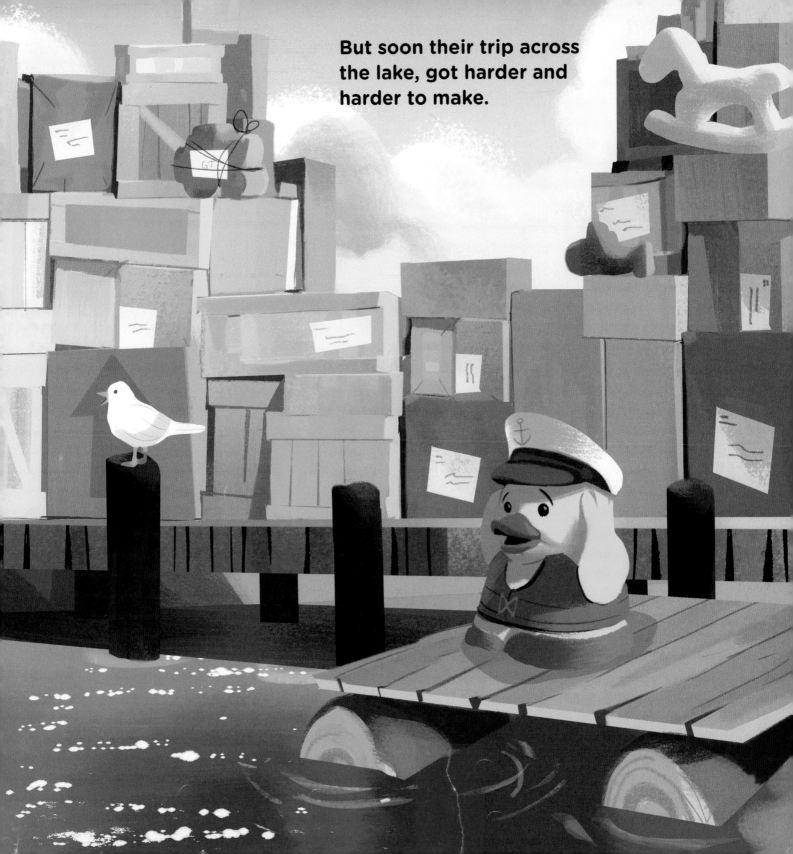

But soon their trip across the lake, got harder and harder to make.

Davey was beat, "I can't feel my feet.
This is a total disaster!

The boxes were plenty, but now there's too many.
How can we ever go faster?"

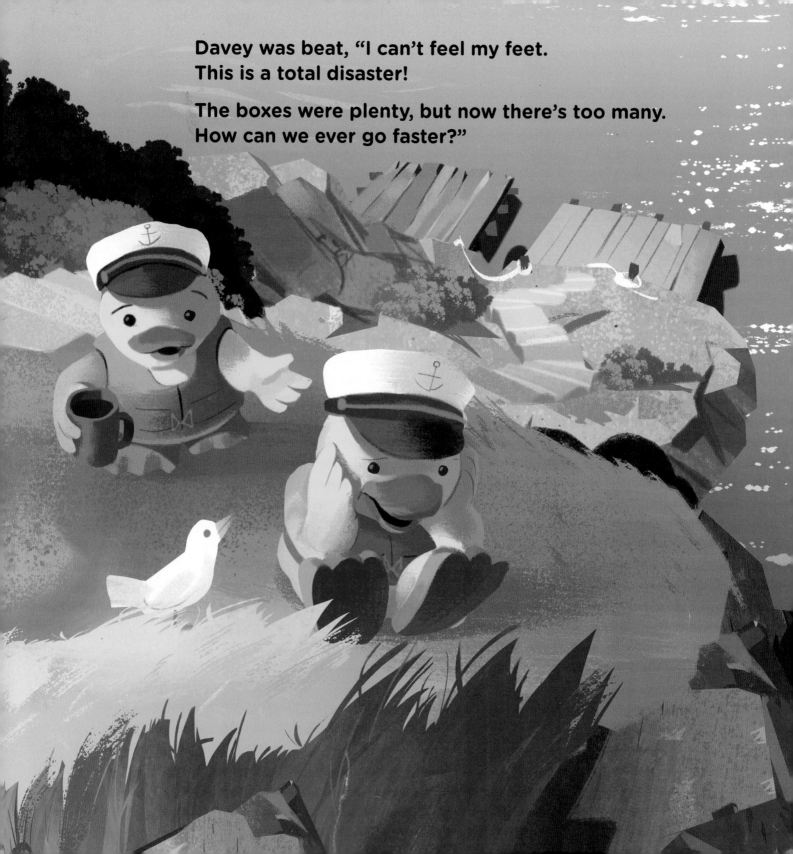

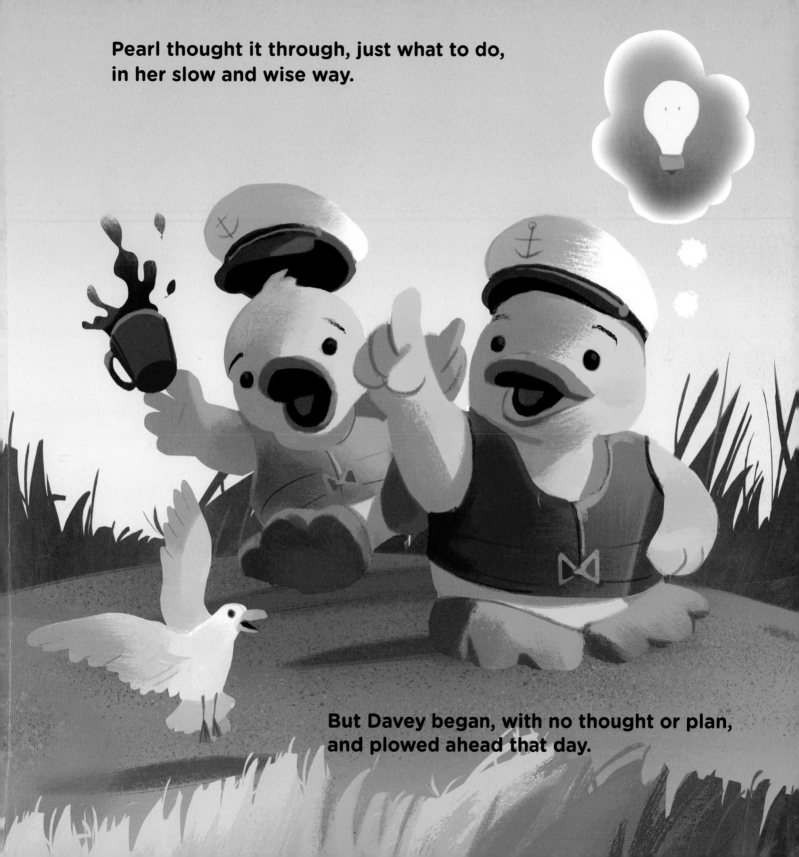

Pearl thought it through, just what to do,
in her slow and wise way.

But Davey began, with no thought or plan,
and plowed ahead that day.

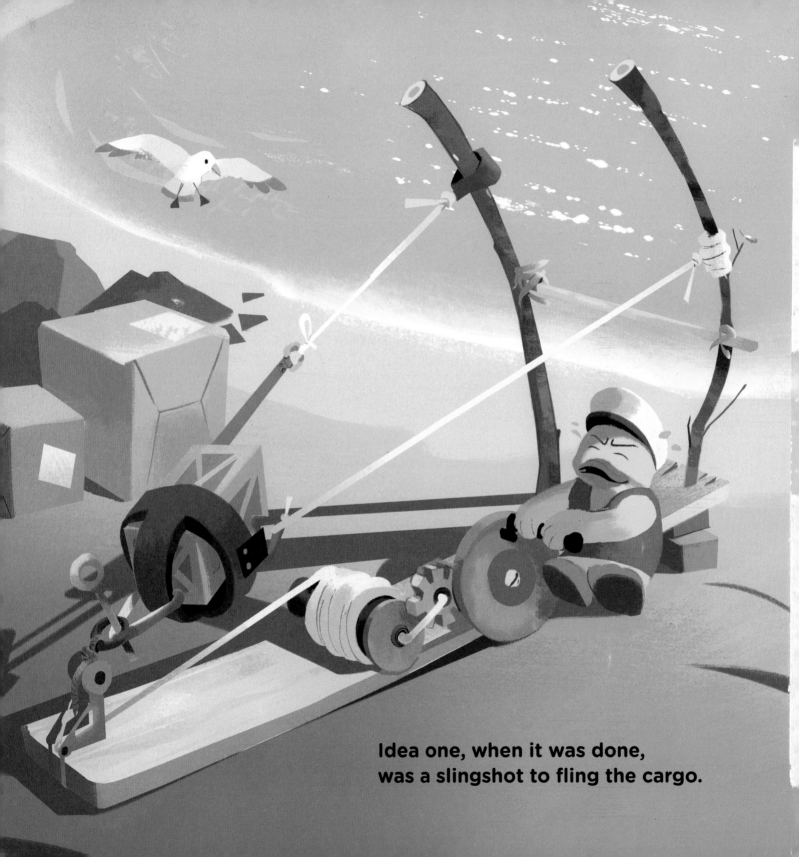

Idea one, when it was done,
was a slingshot to fling the cargo.

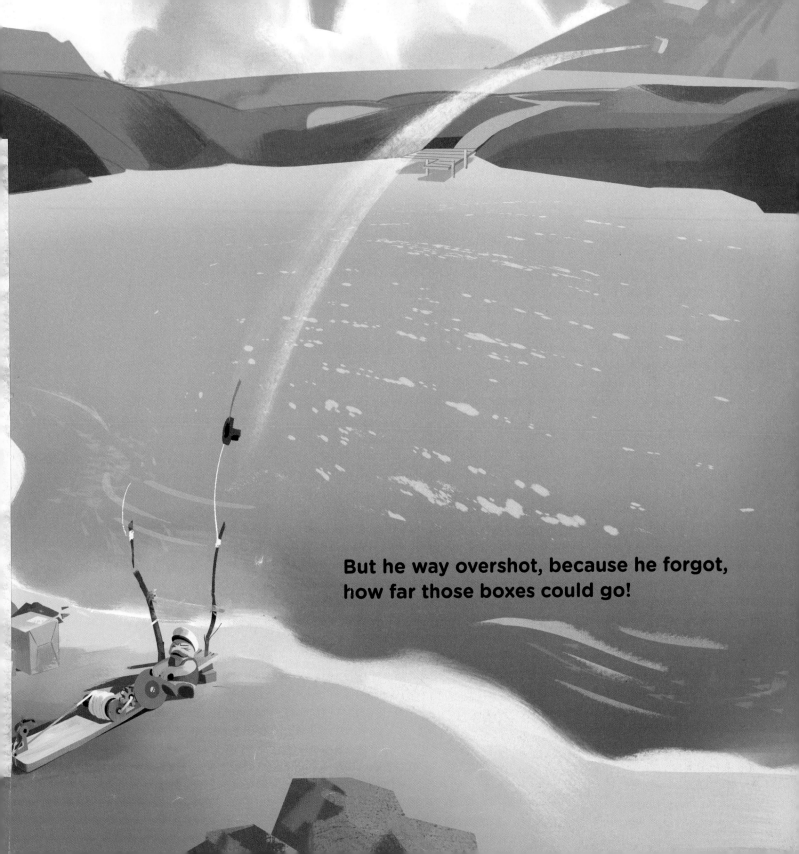

But he way overshot, because he forgot,
how far those boxes could go!

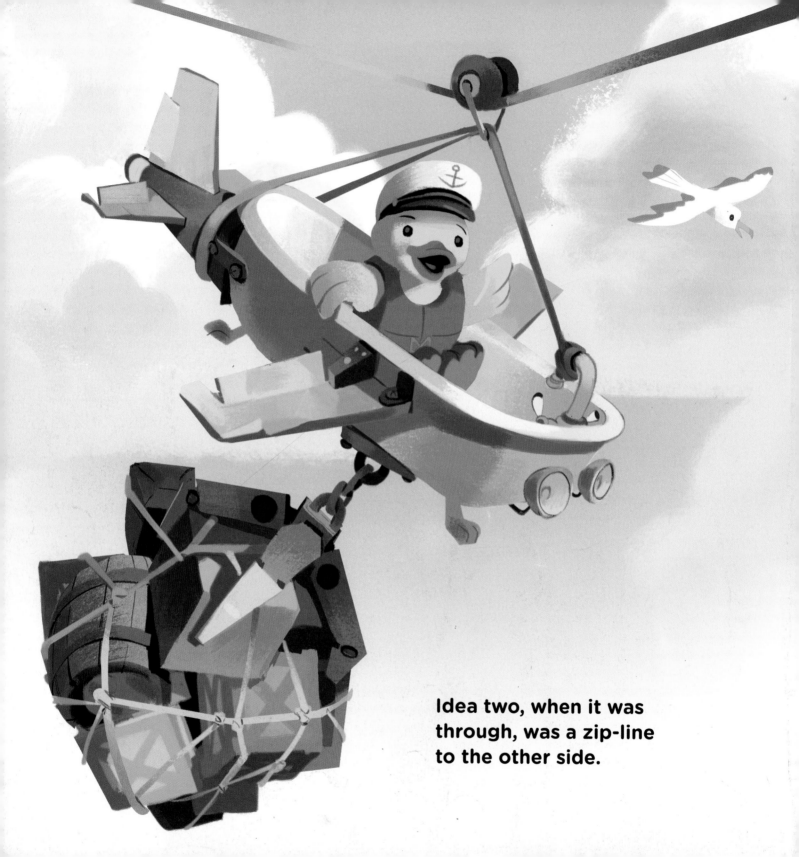

Idea two, when it was
through, was a zip-line
to the other side.

But Davey just dragged,
and the cargo just sagged,
then the zip-line came untied.

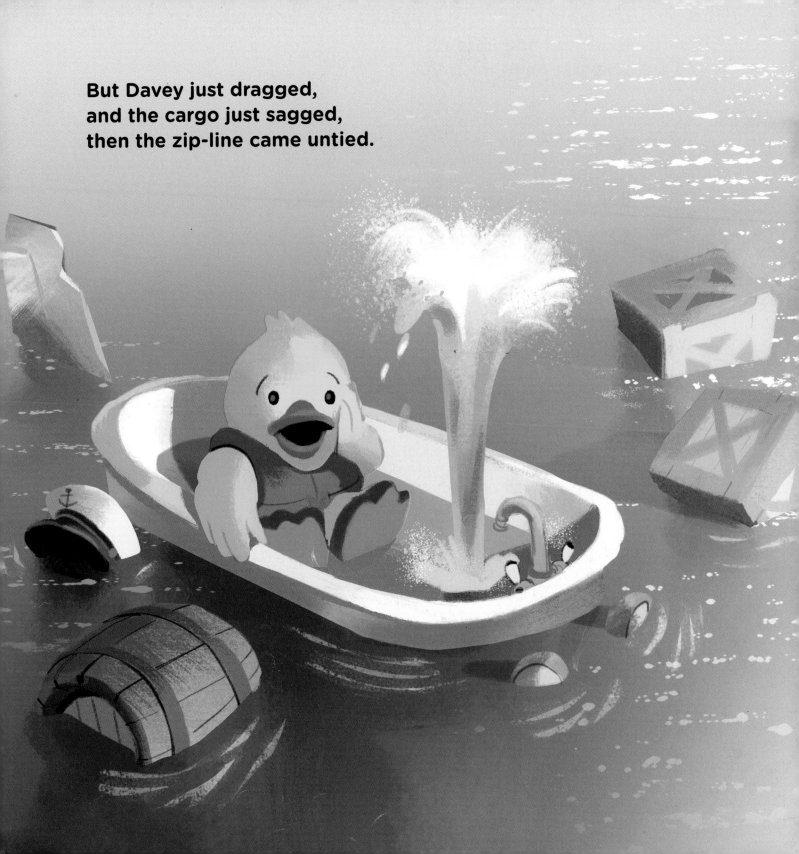

Idea three, a wild one indeed,
was a wacky paddling machine.

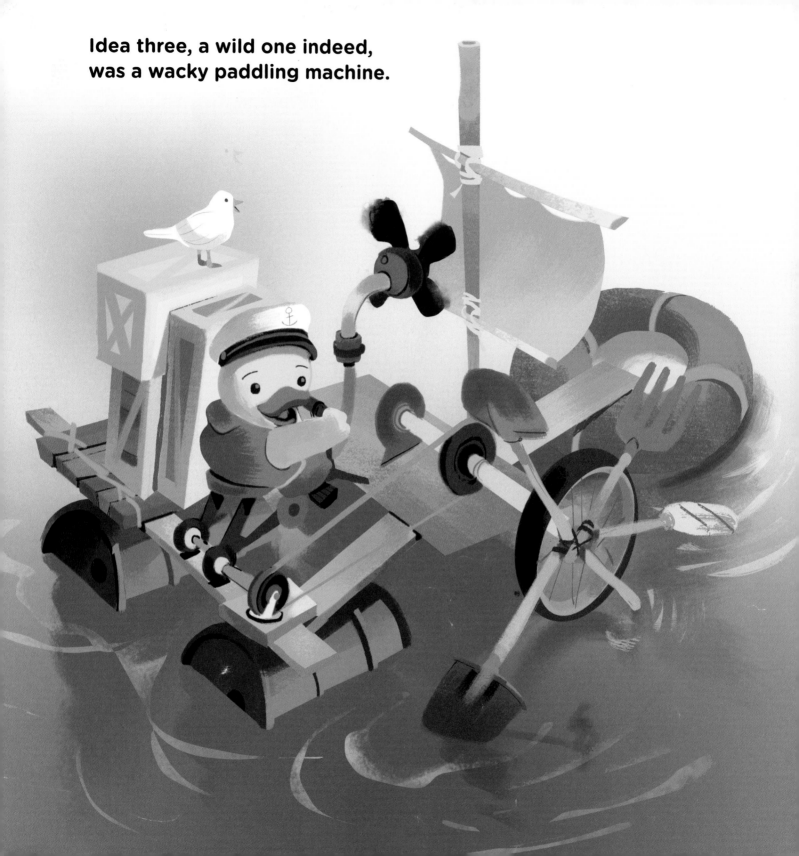

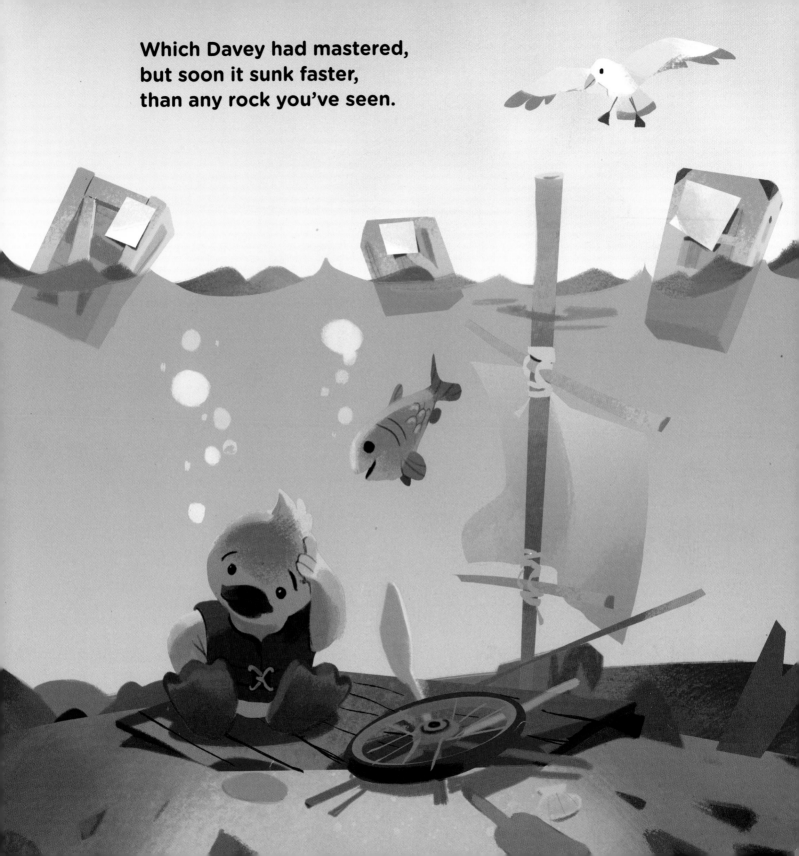

Which Davey had mastered,
but soon it sunk faster,
than any rock you've seen.

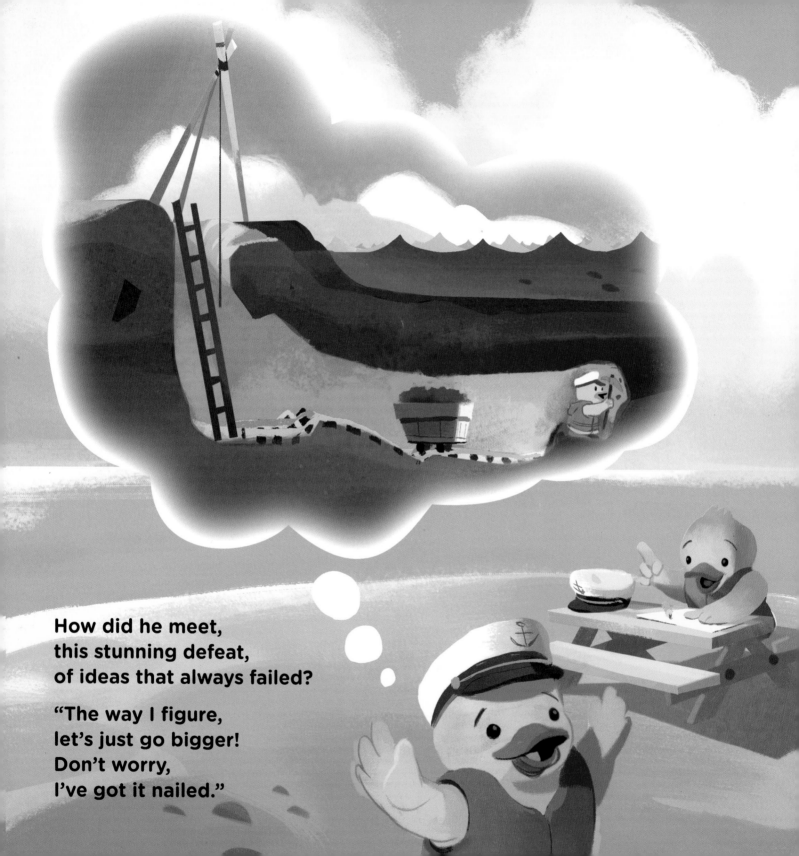

How did he meet,
this stunning defeat,
of ideas that always failed?

"The way I figure,
let's just go bigger!
Don't worry,
I've got it nailed."

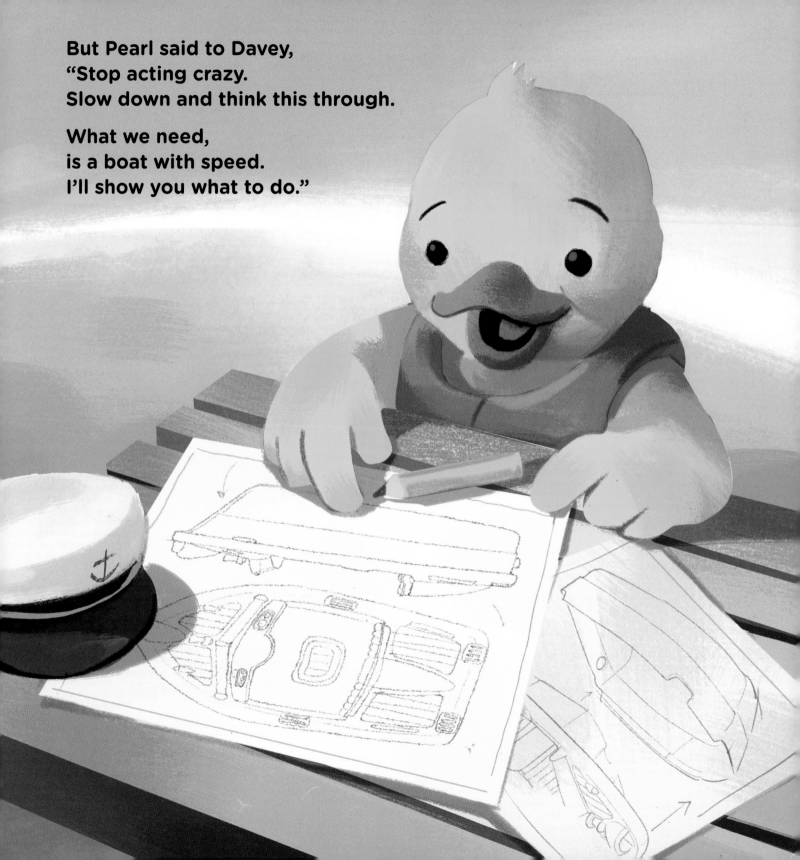

But Pearl said to Davey,
"Stop acting crazy.
Slow down and think this through.

What we need,
is a boat with speed.
I'll show you what to do."

And so they began, to work from her plan,
with Pearl at Davey's side.

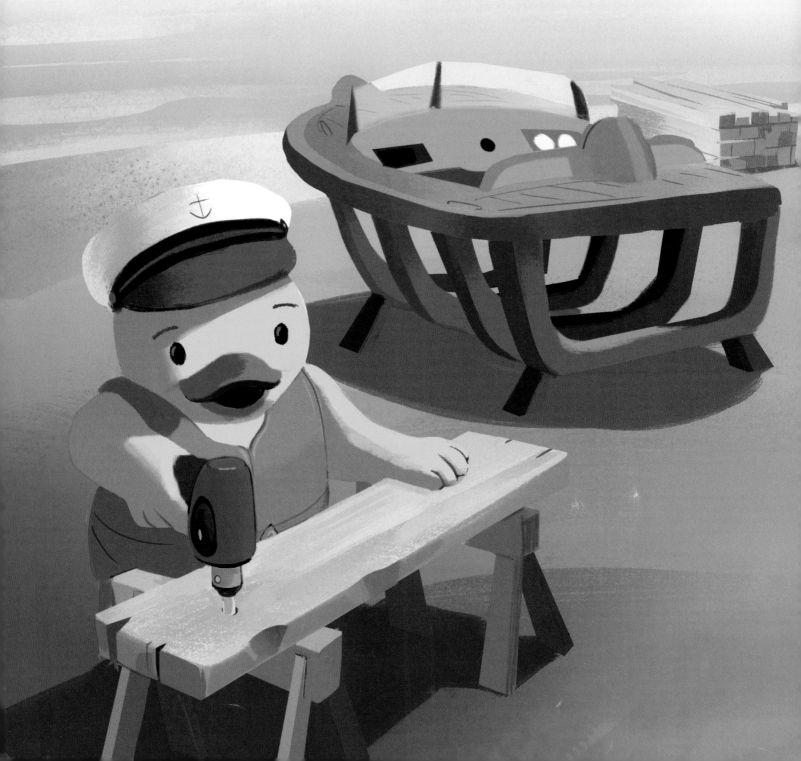

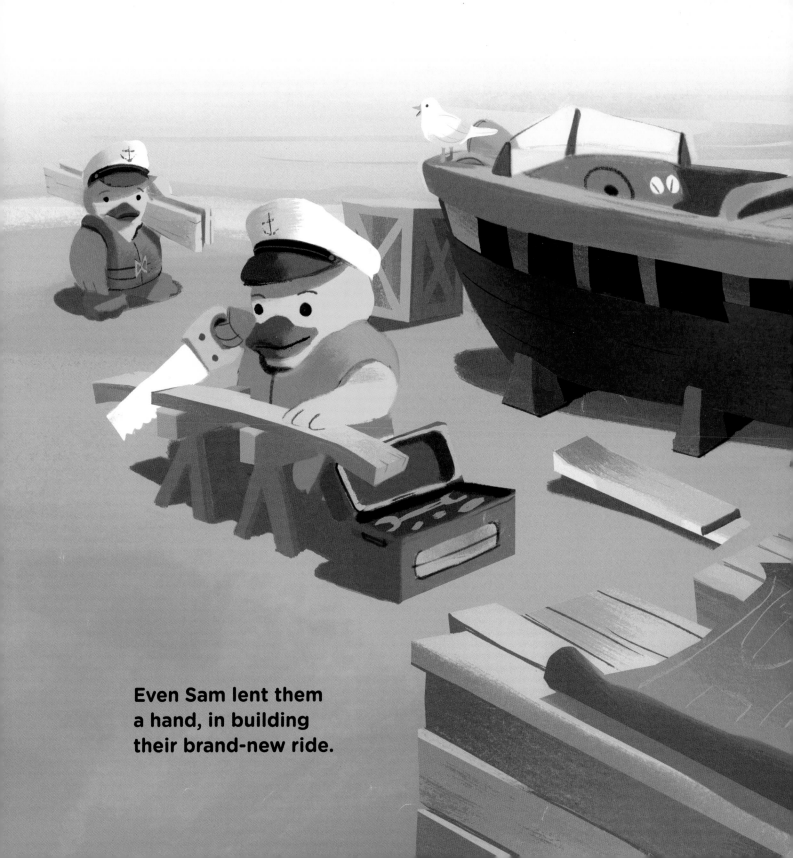

Even Sam lent them
a hand, in building
their brand-new ride.

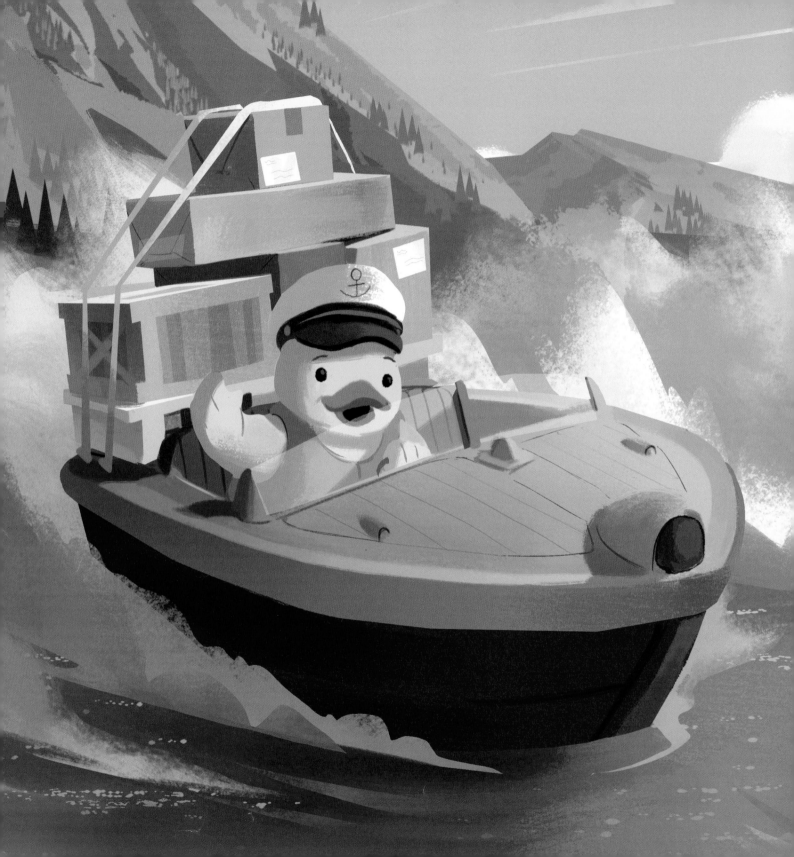

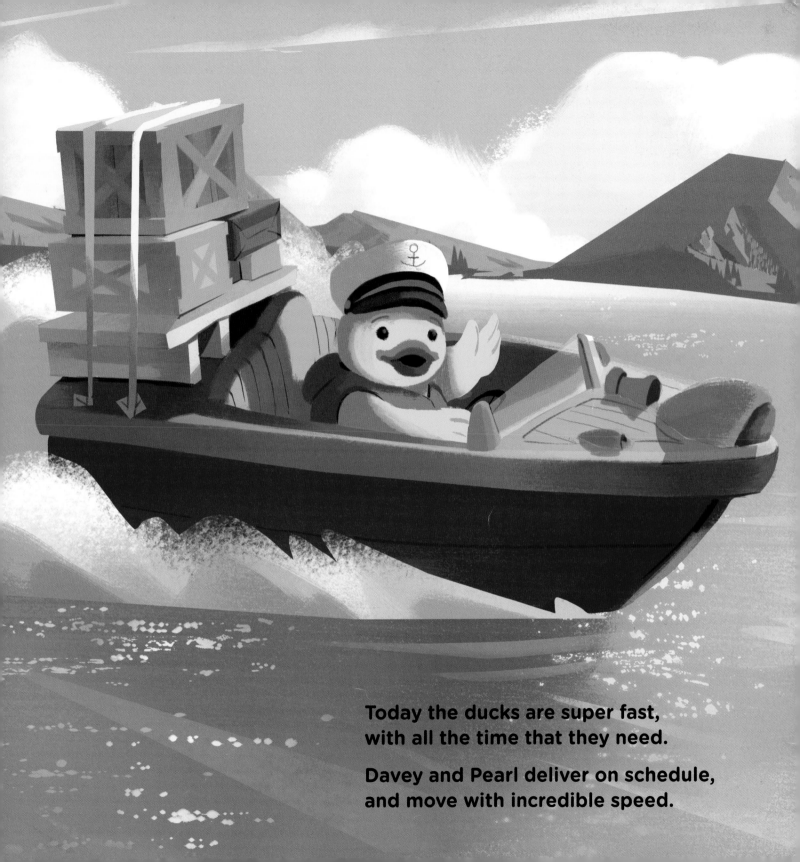

Today the ducks are super fast,
with all the time that they need.

Davey and Pearl deliver on schedule,
and move with incredible speed.

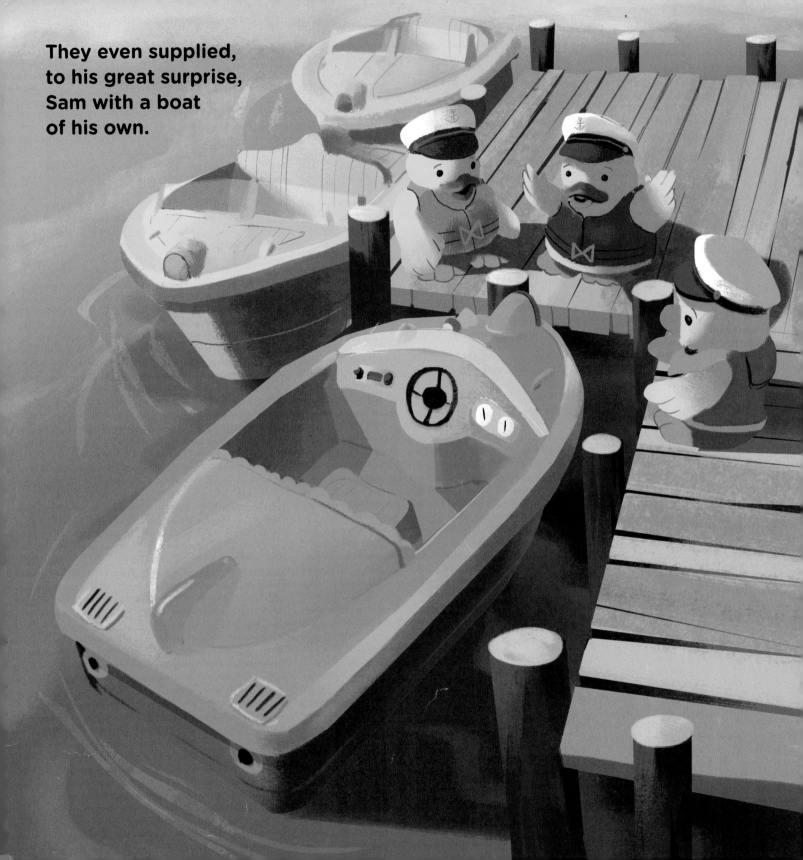

They even supplied,
to his great surprise,
Sam with a boat
of his own.

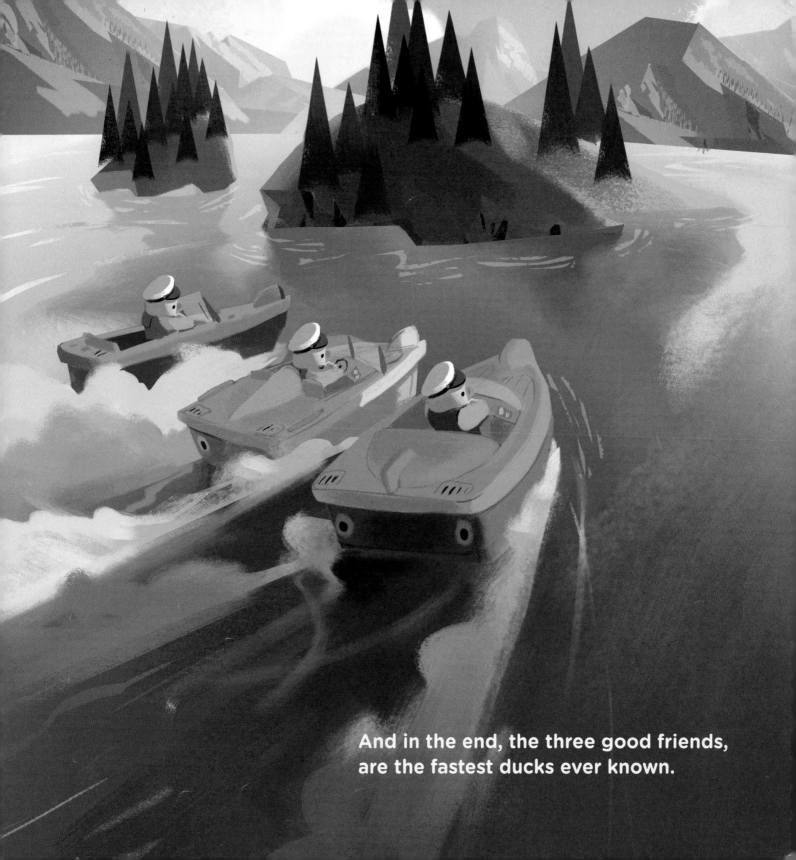

And in the end, the three good friends,
are the fastest ducks ever known.

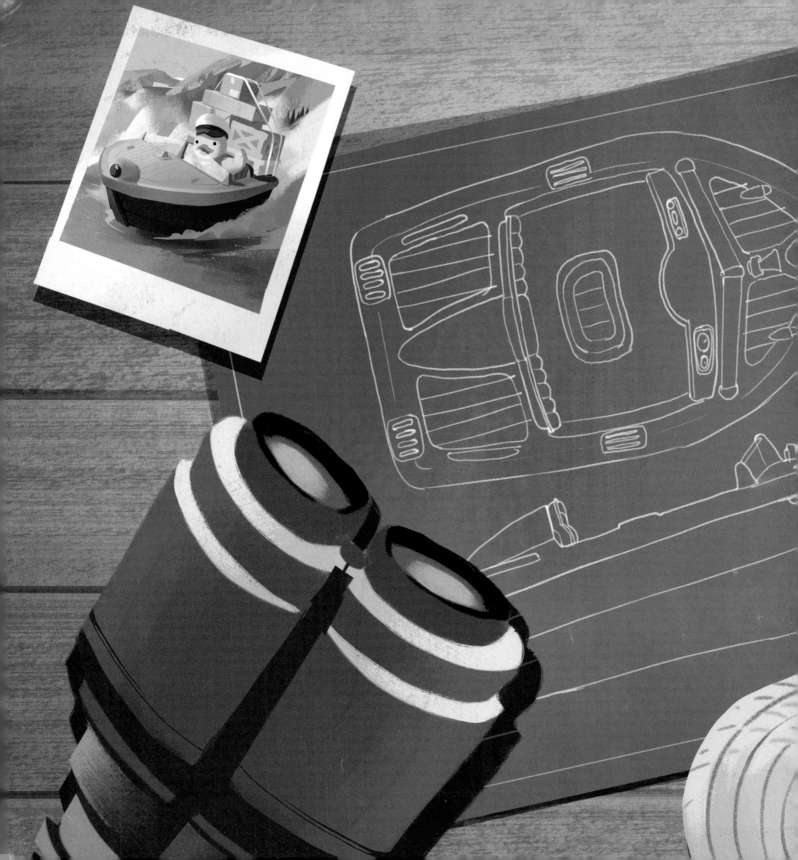